Sheila Phillips

MEMORIES
Of
LOVE and LOSS

Sheila Phillips

MEMORIES
Of
LOVE and LOSS

With a lifelong passion for creative writing, Sheila has gained most of her inspiration from everyday life working as a nurse in healthcare, education and senior management and also as an academic management consultant and associate lecturer in business studies.

Sheila has undertaken voluntary work throughout her life as a Samaritan, Justice of the Peace, Hospital Governor and a consumer researcher at a local BBC radio station. This has given her a wider perspective on human emotion.

Observing people as they go about their daily life has also offered her the privilege of ensuring that their struggles have not gone unnoticed. It is indeed an honour to share this raw emotion through her endearing and thought provoking poetry.

Kindle Direct Publishing
Amazon

Copyright © Sheila Phillips 2025

Sheila Phillips has asserted her right under the Copyright, Designs and Patents Act 1988 to be identified as the author of this work.

ISBN 9798265722003

Printed and bound by Kindle Direct Publishing
http://kdp.amazon.com

Dedicated to the memory of Barbara, Arthur and little Alex

Always in our hearts

'Do not cry because they are past!
Smile because they once were!'

Ludwig Jacobowski

Published in a German Literary Journal

'Das Magazin fur Litteratur' 1899

CONTENTS

Did you see me?
Every moment
An ode to sadness
Angel Whispers
Grief
Untouchable world
A missed life
Turkish delight in Kibris
Ode to Jack the cat
The stage
Going home to Scotland
Was it a dream?
Springtime in Toledo (USA)
Some other life
Candles on Barra
Island life
Bernie's night time visitor
Spring, joy and hope
Because of you
Epitaph

DID YOU SEE ME?

Were you part of my life?
All those years ago?
Affinity broken, transcending our lives
Moving ever forward
Train like, through stations of experience
Damaged by broken promises
Destroyed by broken dreams
Despair, when will your cloak
Lift from my heart?

EVERY MOMENT

Every moment, I learn
To love, to live, to forget
Every moment, I look
Forward, not now, not past
Power to change that to come
Power to let go

AN ODE TO SADNESS

To close my eyes
And drift
Towards a dream
Which is you

Dark clouds
Emptying their tears
Of sadness
Of pain

Soon our lips will touch
Your soft fingers
Clasped in mine
No more to go

Stay close to me
Through the pain and sadness
Making each day a joy
I am whole with you

ANGEL WHISPERS

An angel touched my heart today
With softness, gentleness she caressed
Me until I felt a joy in my fate
Sadness extinguished, this is meant

Her gossamer wings lifted me high,
Higher than the earthly winds
She held me close until peace was mine
Forget your unrest, in life make amends

An angel touched my soul today
How fortunate fate interlocked our hearts
Angels are lightening my way
Now and for the rest of my days

GRIEF

Like a black cloud
Waiting to shed its tears
Of sadness, hopelessness and more
Making me peruse my catalogue of fears

When will this pain subside?
Death how long do you stalk me?
Images of the dying moment
Pervade my waking and sleeping hours.

UNTOUCHABLE WORLD

Like a majestic condor soaring high in the fall sky
Like a butterfly flitting and kissing the summer blossom
Life is not constant but moves from side to side
As we seek to capture the very essence of awesome

Let me peak into your amazing untouchable world
With beautiful words, unseen places and senses unreal
Guide me to a land full of magic as yet unfurled
So that one day we will no longer conceal.

Touch me with your fragrant, perfumed aromas
So that I too can soar to a land full of joy and hope
Shower a cascade of warmth like a hazy summer
When carefree thoughts fill my life in a kaleidoscope

Within the mundane lies beauty, perfection and more
Look and experience this wonderful existence
Take me on a journey to a life I could adore
Break down this immeasurable and vast distance.

A MISSED LIFE

Oh my soul, oh my pain
Heartfelt, a knife in my side
Like a glorious rose petal
Velvet to touch.

Where is that love
I need so much?
Gone forever
Hold me, touch me.

Your very essence fills my soul
Oblivious to all around,
My love is yours until eternity
I wait for death
And peace for evermore.

TURKISH DELIGHT IN KIBRIS

Burlesque, statuesque, Arabesque
Jazzy cushions, crazy rugs
A heart of Middle Eastern dress
How beautiful you look in this world of mediocrity.

Not for you half-stolen measures
Amid the palm trees and aroma-laden jasmine
A home built around a hundred treasures
Of memories new, old and untold.

Arabesque, statuesque, burlesque
How glorious your encompassing comforts
Stand tall 'til your walls are laid to rest
As new tears, joys and sorrows are made.

ODE TO JACK THE CAT

Jack I saw you today
My heart skipped a beat
'I'm here; see me, come and play
No more the sadness nor to weep'

'Yes it's me your life companion
Watching from above over you'
Is it real or am I imagining
The tears in my eyes shade my view

And the tears in my heart remain
Like a dagger driven into my very soul
My love for you Jack will not wane
You're gone and I'm totally alone.

THE STAGE

Look at me, what do you see?
It's not what I am, nor what appears to be
I'm really quite different
From how I may seem
For life's a big act
To fulfill an expected dream

Yet the dream of life
Is not how it should be
The life we lead must be more real
Come, be yourself
Can't you see?
I wish I were me………..

GOING HOME (TO SCOTLAND)

I shouldered a kind of burden
Leaving behind the Tay
My bonnie wee lassies cried
I cried, for myself and them

I yearn for a kind of freedom
Leaving behind the Mersey
My bonnie wee lassies
Will smile, will I?

Tears glistened silently
Then and now
For wisdom is a burden
And freedom has a price

WAS IT A DREAM?

Times spent close to your heart.
Warm loving kisses
Spirits touching
Thoughts locking
The eternity of time motionless
Suspended in timelessness
The softness
Of touch and you
The loving warm glow
Held closely in your arms
Special feeling
Precious moments
Real yet unreal
Yes, it was a dream

SPRINGTIME IN TOLEDO

Oh blossom trees open your sleepy eyes
Feel the warm sunshine pressing against your leaves
Spring flowers blooming where snow once laid
Hold this moment with joy not tears.

The sound of wind chimes teased by spring breezes
Listen, the angels dance along the gossamer winds
Gone are the days when the whole world freezes
Capture this enchanting moment with dear and blessed friends

Oh Toledo spring, good-bye until we meet again
With renewed hope in my heart I will return
There is much to do and much to attain
But I will never forget the joys I have learned

In the beautiful Toledo spring.

SOME OTHER LIFE

The briefest moment in time
Betwixt yesterday and tomorrow
The coolest breeze across our faces
When shared tenderness was mine

Desolation forgotten and abandoned
To the mists of memory.
A kaleidoscope of rainbow threads
Between us woven and fastened

Raindrops shared through embrace
Like a potent solution
Joining our spirits as one.
Once more let me touch your face

If only you knew the pain
Of a dying love,
Would you retrace yesterday?
Will you come back again?

CANDLES ON BARRA

I remember those days granddad
With fierce winds blowing
Across mountains and lochs
Rattling the shutters
With dancing rain
Plucked from the ocean
Cascaded upon the roof.

Candles flickering
As if nervously jittering
In anticipation of extinction
My love for you shines
As brightly as the candles today
Radiant in my bedroom
Like a row of living pearls.

How I wish
For those Island days of yesteryear............

Island Life – Then and Now (Thoughts on the Battle of Leros WW2)

See the seagulls swoop so low?
As if in mock battle
Like aeroplanes in full flow
From a bygone, forgotten past

This land so full of exquisiteness
The smell of blossom-laden trees
The sounds of local folk
Some dressed in black, for tears

The sights of blue and white houses
Churches, tiny shops and more
Hide the horrors which once
Befell this paradise, yes war

BERNIE'S NIGHT TIME VISITOR

Tap, tap, what is that sound?

Bernie awakes and looks all around

'It's still dark I should be asleep,

Oh it's louder I must take a peak'.

Tap, tap, tap, 'it's on my window,

Do you want to come in?' he whispers low

To a big orange and white kitty

'Oh my' Bernie laughs, 'you look so pretty'.

'And where is your mummy, your daddy too?

You frightened me so; I didn't know it was you'

'I want to snuggle up' Ginger replied

With that Bernie and his friend cosied up side by side.

SPRING JOY AND HOPE

I am nowhere, but everywhere
Buried deep in your heart
Though we're apart
The Spring blossoms a reminder
Of the cycle of life.

Dying, re-birth, renew
My thoughts are with you
As we tread this lonely path
'Primavera' it is
Yes, Spring is here.

BECAUSE OF YOU

You made me smile

When I couldn't smile

You made me happy

When life was sad

Your kindness shone through

Amid our frenetic life

Without you, it's full of strife

My existence, so enhanced

Because of you……….

EPITAPH

Two kindred spirits caught in time
Joined complete as one
Precious moments left behind
Dispersed, with time, now gone.

How many of us have yearned for the past when life felt complete and whole surrounded by those we loved? The loss of loved ones, animals and close friends. The loss of identity, self esteem, lifestyle and self respect can engender so many feelings of loneliness, solitude and hopelessness.

This pocket book Anthology seeks to provide a poignant reminder of how love and loss are uniquely intertwined. Beautiful poetry offering solace during times of sad reflection and giving comfort and greater understanding to those who may be suffering.

Printed in Dunstable, United Kingdom